LOW-BUDGET TYPE 2 DIABETES COOKBOOK FOR BEGINNERS

The Ultimate Guide To Healthy, Wallet-Friendly, Low-Carb, Low-Sugar, Diabetes Diet Recipes, With A 31-Day Meal Plan

Marcus Baron

Table of Contents

COPYRIGHT © 2023

CHAPTER ONE

Introduction to Low-Budget Diabetic Cooking

Living with type 2 diabetes requires careful management of diet and lifestyle to maintain optimal health. One significant aspect of managing diabetes is adhering to a healthy diet, which can sometimes be challenging, especially for those on a tight budget. However, with the right knowledge and strategies, it's possible to prepare nutritious and delicious meals without breaking the bank. This guide aims to provide a comprehensive overview of low-budget diabetic cooking, covering the importance of budget-friendly meals for type 2 diabetes, tips for cooking healthy meals on a tight budget, and essential pantry staples for affordable diabetic cooking.

Understanding the Importance of Budget-Friendly Meals for Type 2 Diabetes

Type 2 diabetes is a chronic condition characterized by insulin resistance, where the body's cells don't respond effectively to insulin. This leads to high blood sugar levels, which can have serious health consequences if not properly managed. Diet plays a crucial role in managing type 2 diabetes, as certain foods can affect blood sugar levels more than others.

For individuals with type 2 diabetes, it's essential to focus on consuming a balanced diet that includes plenty of fruits, vegetables, whole grains, lean proteins, and healthy fats while limiting refined sugars, saturated fats, and processed foods. However, eating healthily can sometimes be expensive, especially for those on limited incomes.

Budget-friendly meals for type 2 diabetes are important for several reasons:

1. **Cost-Effective Management**: Managing type 2 diabetes can be expensive, with costs associated with medications, supplies, and healthcare visits. By preparing budget-friendly meals, individuals can save money on groceries, reducing overall healthcare costs.

2. **Promotes Long-Term Health**: Eating a healthy diet is essential for managing blood sugar levels, reducing the risk of complications associated with type 2 diabetes, such as heart disease, stroke, and nerve damage. Budget-friendly meals allow individuals to maintain a nutritious diet without financial strain, promoting better long-term health outcomes.

3. **Encourages Adherence to Dietary Guidelines**: Many individuals with type 2 diabetes struggle to adhere to dietary recommendations due to the perceived cost of healthy foods. By offering budget-friendly meal options, individuals are more likely to follow dietary guidelines, leading to better diabetes management and improved overall well-being.

Tips for Cooking Healthy Meals on a Tight Budget

Cooking healthy meals on a tight budget requires careful planning, smart shopping, and creative cooking techniques. Here are some practical tips to help individuals with type 2 diabetes prepare nutritious meals without overspending:

1. **Plan Meals in Advance**: Before heading to the grocery store, take the time to plan your meals for the week. Consider incorporating affordable ingredients such as beans, lentils, rice, and seasonal vegetables into your meal plan. Planning ahead helps avoid impulse purchases and ensures you have all the necessary ingredients on hand.

2. **Shop Smart**: When shopping for groceries, look for sales, discounts, and bulk deals to maximize your savings. Consider purchasing store-brand items, which are often cheaper than name brands but comparable in quality. Additionally, buying in bulk can help lower the cost per serving, especially for staples like rice, pasta, and canned goods.

3. **Embrace Plant-Based Proteins**: Protein is an essential nutrient for individuals with type 2 diabetes, but it doesn't have to break the bank. Plant-based sources of protein, such as beans, lentils, tofu, and eggs, are generally more affordable than meat and poultry. Incorporating these...

Essential Pantry Staples for Affordable Diabetic Cooking

Stocking your pantry with essential ingredients is key to preparing affordable and nutritious meals for type 2 diabetes. Having a well-stocked pantry ensures you have the basics on hand to whip up delicious dishes without having to make frequent trips to the grocery store. Here are some essential pantry staples for affordable diabetic cooking:

1. **Whole Grains**: Whole grains are rich in fiber and nutrients, making them an excellent choice for individuals with type 2 diabetes. Stock up on staples like brown rice, quinoa, oats, and whole wheat pasta. These grains can serve as the foundation for many budget-friendly meals, such as stir-fries, salads, and grain bowls.

2. **Legumes**: Beans, lentils, and chickpeas are affordable sources of protein and fiber that can help stabilize blood sugar levels. Keep a variety of canned and dried legumes in your pantry to add to soups, stews, salads, and...

By incorporating these pantry staples into your cooking routine, you can prepare delicious and nutritious meals for type 2 diabetes without breaking the bank. With a little planning and creativity, eating healthily on a tight budget is entirely achievable.

CHAPTER TWO

Shopping Smart on a Budget

In today's economy, many individuals and families are looking for ways to stretch their budgets further, and one area where significant savings can be made is on groceries. Smart shopping involves not only finding the best deals but also ensuring that you're making healthy choices for you and your family. This guide explores strategies for saving money on groceries without sacrificing nutrition, tips for meal planning to stretch your budget further, and making the most of sales, coupons, and discounts.

Strategies for Saving Money on Groceries Without Sacrificing Nutrition

1. **Shop Seasonally**: Seasonal produce is often fresher and more affordable than out-of-season options. Fruits and vegetables that are in season are typically abundant, leading to lower prices. Additionally, local farmers' markets may offer discounts on seasonal produce, providing an opportunity to support local growers while saving money.

2. **Buy in Bulk**: Purchasing items in bulk can lead to significant savings over time, especially for pantry staples like rice, pasta, beans, and canned goods. Look for bulk bins at grocery stores or consider joining a warehouse club where you can buy larger quantities at lower prices. Just be sure to...

Tips for Meal Planning to Stretch Your Budget Further

1. **Plan Meals Based on Sales**: Take advantage of weekly sales flyers from grocery stores to plan your meals around discounted items. If chicken breast is on sale, plan several

meals that incorporate chicken as the main protein. By building your meal plan around sale items, you can save money while still enjoying nutritious meals.

2. **Use Leftovers Wisely**: Leftovers can be a valuable resource for stretching your food budget further. When cooking meals, intentionally make extra servings to have leftovers for future meals. Get creative with repurposing leftovers into new dishes, such as turning roasted vegetables into a...

Making the Most of Sales, Coupons, and Discounts

1. **Sign Up for Loyalty Programs**: Many grocery stores offer loyalty programs that provide discounts, coupons, and special offers to members. Sign up for these programs to take advantage of exclusive savings opportunities. Some programs also offer personalized discounts based on your purchasing history, allowing you to save money on items you regularly buy.

2. **Clip Coupons**: Traditional paper coupons may seem old-fashioned, but they can still lead to significant savings on groceries. Look for coupons in newspapers, magazines, and coupon websites, and clip them for items you regularly purchase. Additionally, many grocery stores offer digital coupons that can be loaded directly onto your loyalty card for easy...

By employing these strategies and tips, you can shop smart on a budget without sacrificing nutrition or flavor. With a little planning and creativity, you can stretch your food dollars further while still enjoying delicious and nutritious meals.

CHAPTER THREE

Quick and Easy Breakfasts

Breakfast is often hailed as the most important meal of the day, providing the energy and nutrients needed to kickstart your morning. However, busy schedules and limited time can make it challenging to prepare a nutritious breakfast. This guide offers simple and budget-friendly breakfast ideas that are quick to make and use affordable ingredients. From hearty oatmeal variations to egg-based dishes, these recipes will help you start your day off right without breaking the bank.

Simple Breakfast Recipes Using Affordable Ingredients

1. **Banana Oat Pancakes**:

- Ingredients:

    - 1 ripe banana, mashed

    - 1 egg

    - 1/2 cup rolled oats

    - 1/2 teaspoon cinnamon

    - Optional toppings: sliced bananas, berries, maple syrup

- Instructions:

1. In a bowl, combine mashed banana, egg, rolled oats, and cinnamon.

2. Heat a non-stick skillet over medium heat and lightly coat with cooking spray.

3. Pour batter onto the skillet to form pancakes and cook until bubbles form on the surface.

4. Flip and cook for another 1-2 minutes until golden brown.

5. Serve hot with your favorite toppings.

2. **Yogurt Parfait**:

- Ingredients:

  - Greek yogurt

  - Granola

  - Fresh fruit (e.g., berries, sliced bananas)

  - Honey or maple syrup (optional)

- Instructions:

1. In a glass or bowl, layer Greek yogurt, granola, and fresh fruit.

2. Drizzle with honey or maple syrup if desired.

3. Repeat layers until the glass or bowl is filled.

4. Serve immediately or refrigerate for later.

Budget-Friendly Oatmeal Variations for a Filling Start to the Day

1. **Classic Oatmeal**:

   - Ingredients:

     - 1/2 cup rolled oats

     - 1 cup water or milk

     - Pinch of salt

     - Optional toppings: sliced bananas, berries, nuts, honey or maple syrup

- Instructions:

1.   In a saucepan, bring water or milk to a boil.

2.   Stir in rolled oats and salt, reduce heat to low, and simmer for 5 minutes, stirring occasionally.

3.   Remove from heat and let it sit for a minute before serving.

4.   Top with your favorite toppings and enjoy.

2. Apple Cinnamon Oatmeal:

- Ingredients:

    - 1/2 cup rolled oats

    - 1 cup water or milk

    - 1/2 apple, diced

    - 1/2 teaspoon cinnamon

    - Optional toppings: sliced apples, chopped nuts, honey or maple syrup

- Instructions:

1.   In a saucepan, combine water or milk, rolled oats, diced apple, and cinnamon.

2.   Bring to a boil, then reduce heat to low and simmer for 5 minutes, stirring occasionally.

3.   Remove from heat and let it sit for a minute before serving.

4.   Top with additional sliced apples, chopped nuts, and a drizzle of honey or maple syrup if desired.

Egg-Based Breakfast Dishes That Won't Break the Bank

1. **Vegetable Frittata**:

- Ingredients:

    - Eggs

    - Assorted vegetables (e.g., bell peppers, onions, spinach)

    - Cheese (optional)

    - Salt and pepper to taste

- Instructions:

1.   Preheat oven to 350°F (175°C).

2.   In a skillet, sauté vegetables until tender.

3.   In a bowl, beat eggs and season with salt and pepper.

4.   Pour beaten eggs over the vegetables in the skillet.

5.   Cook on the stovetop for a few minutes until the edges begin to set.

6. Sprinkle cheese on top (if using) and transfer the skillet to the oven.

7. Bake for 10-12 minutes or until the eggs are set and the top is golden brown.

8. Slice into wedges and serve hot.

2. **Scrambled Egg Wraps**:

- Ingredients:

  - Eggs

  - Tortillas

  - Optional fillings: diced tomatoes, avocado, cheese, salsa

- Instructions:

1. In a bowl, beat eggs and season with salt and pepper.

2. Heat a non-stick skillet over medium heat and pour in beaten eggs.

3. Cook, stirring occasionally, until the eggs are scrambled and cooked through.

4. Warm tortillas in the skillet or microwave.

5. Place scrambled eggs onto the center of each tortilla and add desired fillings.

6.   Fold in the sides of the tortilla and roll it up tightly.

7.   Serve immediately or wrap in foil for an on-the-go breakfast.

These quick and easy breakfast recipes are perfect for busy mornings and won't put a strain on your wallet. With simple ingredients and minimal preparation time, you can enjoy a nutritious and satisfying breakfast without breaking the bank.

CHAPTER FOUR

Budget-Friendly Lunches

Lunchtime is an opportunity to refuel and recharge during a busy day, but it doesn't have to break the bank. With a bit of creativity and strategic planning, you can enjoy delicious and satisfying lunches without spending a fortune. This guide offers budget-friendly lunch ideas, including affordable salad and sandwich options, creative ways to use leftovers, and hearty soups and stews made with inexpensive ingredients.

Affordable Salad and Sandwich Ideas for Satisfying Midday Meals

1. **Greek Salad with Chickpeas:**

   - Ingredients:

     - Mixed greens

     - Cucumber, diced

     - Cherry tomatoes, halved

     - Red onion, thinly sliced

     - Canned chickpeas, drained and rinsed

     - Feta cheese, crumbled

     - Kalamata olives

     - Greek dressing (olive oil, lemon juice, garlic, oregano)

   - Instructions:

1. In a large bowl, combine mixed greens, cucumber, cherry tomatoes, red onion, chickpeas, feta cheese, and olives.

2. Drizzle with Greek dressing and toss to coat.

3.   Serve immediately as a light and refreshing lunch option.

2. **Turkey and Avocado Wrap**:

- Ingredients:
    - Whole wheat tortilla
    - Sliced turkey breast
    - Avocado, sliced
    - Lettuce
    - Tomato, sliced
    - Mustard or mayo (optional)
- Instructions:

1.   Lay the tortilla flat and layer with turkey slices, avocado, lettuce, and tomato.

2.   Spread mustard or mayo on top if desired.

3.   Roll up the tortilla tightly and slice in half.

4.   Serve immediately or wrap in foil for a portable lunch option.

Creative Ways to Use Leftovers for Quick and Cheap Lunches

1. **Quinoa Salad with Roasted Vegetables**:

- Ingredients:
    - Cooked quinoa

- Assorted roasted vegetables (e.g., bell peppers, zucchini, eggplant)

- Chickpeas

- Feta cheese (optional)

- Balsamic vinaigrette

- Instructions:

1. In a bowl, combine cooked quinoa, roasted vegetables, and chickpeas.

2. Crumble feta cheese on top if desired.

3. Drizzle with balsamic vinaigrette and toss to coat.

4. Serve chilled or at room temperature for a hearty and nutritious lunch.

2. **Stir-Fry Rice Bowl**:

- Ingredients:

- Cooked rice (white or brown)

- Leftover cooked chicken, beef, or tofu

- Mixed vegetables (e.g., bell peppers, broccoli, carrots)

- Soy sauce or teriyaki sauce

- Sesame seeds (optional)

- Instructions:

1.   In a skillet, stir-fry leftover meat or tofu with mixed vegetables until heated through.

2.   Add cooked rice to the skillet and stir to combine.

3.   Season with soy sauce or teriyaki sauce to taste.

4.   Sprinkle with sesame seeds if desired and serve hot for a quick and satisfying lunch option.

Soups and Stews Made with Inexpensive Ingredients

1. **Vegetable Lentil Soup**:

- Ingredients:

    - Lentils

    - Assorted vegetables (e.g., carrots, celery, onions)

    - Vegetable broth

    - Canned diced tomatoes

    - Garlic, minced

    - Herbs and spices (e.g., thyme, bay leaves, paprika)

- Instructions:

1.   In a large pot, sauté garlic, onions, and carrots until softened.

2.   Add lentils, diced tomatoes, vegetable broth, and herbs/spices to the pot.

3.   Bring to a boil, then reduce heat and simmer for 20-25 minutes until lentils are tender.

4.   Season with salt and pepper to taste and serve hot for a nutritious and satisfying lunch option.

2. **Bean and Vegetable Stew**:

- Ingredients:
    - Assorted beans (e.g., black beans, kidney beans, cannellini beans)
    - Assorted vegetables (e.g., bell peppers, squash, corn)
    - Onion, diced
    - Garlic, minced
    - Vegetable broth
    - Canned diced tomatoes
    - Herbs and spices (e.g., cumin, chili powder, oregano)

- Instructions:

1. In a large pot, sauté garlic and onion until fragrant.

2. Add assorted beans, vegetables, diced tomatoes, vegetable broth, and herbs/spices to the pot.

3. Bring to a boil, then reduce heat and simmer for 15-20 minutes until vegetables are tender.

4. Serve hot with a dollop of Greek yogurt or a sprinkle of cheese for added flavor.

These budget-friendly lunch ideas are perfect for anyone looking to save money without sacrificing flavor or nutrition. With simple ingredients and easy preparation, you can enjoy satisfying midday meals that won't break the bank.

CHAPTER FIVE

Economical Dinners for Every Night

Preparing dinner on a budget doesn't mean sacrificing taste or nutrition. With a little planning and creativity, you can whip up delicious and satisfying meals that won't break the bank. This guide presents a variety of economical dinner ideas, including one-pot meals, meatless options, and slow cooker/instant pot recipes, perfect for every night of the week.

One-Pot Meals That Are Budget-Friendly and Delicious

1. **Vegetable Stir-Fry with Rice**:

   - Ingredients:
     - Assorted vegetables (e.g., bell peppers, broccoli, carrots)
     - Firm tofu or chicken breast, cubed (optional)
     - Soy sauce or teriyaki sauce
     - Cooked rice
     - Sesame seeds (optional)
   - Instructions:

1. In a large skillet or wok, stir-fry vegetables and tofu or chicken (if using) until tender.

2. Add soy sauce or teriyaki sauce to taste and continue cooking until heated through.

3. Serve over cooked rice and sprinkle with sesame seeds if desired for a quick and nutritious dinner option.

2. **Pasta Primavera**:

- Ingredients:

    - Pasta (e.g., spaghetti, penne)

    - Assorted vegetables (e.g., zucchini, cherry tomatoes, spinach)

    - Garlic, minced

    - Olive oil

    - Parmesan cheese (optional)

- Instructions:

1.   Cook pasta according to package instructions until al dente. Drain and set aside.

2.   In a large skillet, sauté minced garlic in olive oil until fragrant.

3.   Add assorted vegetables to the skillet and cook until tender.

4.   Toss cooked pasta with the vegetable mixture and season with salt and pepper to taste.

5.   Serve hot with a sprinkle of Parmesan cheese if desired for a simple and satisfying dinner.

Meatless Dinner Options to Save Money on Protein

1. **Vegetable and Bean Chili**:

    - Ingredients:

- Assorted beans (e.g., kidney beans, black beans, cannellini beans)

- Diced tomatoes

- Onion, diced

- Bell peppers, diced

- Garlic, minced

- Chili powder, cumin, paprika

- Instructions:

1. In a large pot, sauté diced onion and minced garlic until softened.

2. Add diced bell peppers and cook until slightly softened.

3. Stir in assorted beans, diced tomatoes, and spices.

4. Bring to a simmer and cook for 20-30 minutes until flavors are blended and vegetables are tender.

5. Serve hot with your favorite chili toppings, such as shredded cheese, sour cream, and chopped green onions.

2. **Quinoa and Black Bean Burrito Bowl**:

- Ingredients:

- Cooked quinoa

- Canned black beans, drained and rinsed

- Corn kernels

- Salsa

- Avocado, diced

- Cilantro, chopped

- Instructions:

1.   In a bowl, layer cooked quinoa, black beans, corn, salsa, and diced avocado.

2.   Garnish with chopped cilantro and serve hot for a flavorful and protein-packed dinner option.

Slow Cooker and Instant Pot Recipes for Effortless Cooking

1. **Slow Cooker Vegetable Soup**:

- Ingredients:

    - Assorted vegetables (e.g., carrots, celery, potatoes)

    - Vegetable broth

    - Canned diced tomatoes

    - Garlic, minced

    - Herbs and spices (e.g., thyme, rosemary, bay leaves)

- Instructions:

1. Combine chopped vegetables, vegetable broth, canned diced tomatoes, minced garlic, and herbs/spices in a slow cooker.

2. Cook on low for 6-8 hours or high for 3-4 hours until vegetables are tender.

3. Season with salt and pepper to taste and serve hot for a comforting and nourishing dinner.

2. **Instant Pot Lentil Curry**:

- Ingredients:
    - Lentils
    - Assorted vegetables (e.g., onions, bell peppers, tomatoes)
    - Curry powder
    - Coconut milk
    - Vegetable broth
- Instructions:

1. In the Instant Pot, sauté onions, bell peppers, and tomatoes until softened.

2. Stir in lentils, curry powder, coconut milk, and vegetable broth.

3.	Seal the Instant Pot and cook on high pressure for 10 minutes.

4.	Allow natural pressure release for 5 minutes, then manually release any remaining pressure.

5.	Serve hot over rice or with naan bread for a flavorful and satisfying dinner.

These economical dinner ideas offer a variety of options to suit every taste and dietary preference. Whether you're cooking for yourself, your family, or a crowd, these recipes are sure to please without breaking the bank.

CHAPTER SIX

Snacks on a Shoestring Budget

When hunger strikes between meals, having affordable and nutritious snack options on hand can help you stay satisfied without breaking the bank. This guide explores budget-friendly snack ideas using pantry staples, homemade snacks that are low in cost and high in flavor, and convenient snack packs for on-the-go convenience.

Affordable Snack Ideas Using Pantry Staples

1. **Popcorn**:

   - Popcorn kernels are an inexpensive pantry staple that can be popped on the stove or in the microwave. Season with salt, nutritional yeast, or spices for a flavorful snack that's high in fiber and low in calories.

2. **Trail Mix**:

   - Create your own trail mix using a combination of nuts, seeds, dried fruit, and whole grain cereal. Buying these ingredients in bulk allows you to customize your mix while keeping costs low.

3. **Rice Cakes with Toppings**:

   - Rice cakes are a versatile and budget-friendly snack option. Top them with peanut butter and banana slices, hummus and cucumber, or avocado and salsa for a satisfying and nutritious treat.

Homemade Snacks That Are Low in Cost and High in Flavor

1. **Energy Bites**:

   - Combine rolled oats, nut butter, honey or maple syrup, and mix-ins like chocolate chips, dried fruit, or nuts. Roll into bite-sized balls and refrigerate for a quick and portable snack that's packed with protein and fiber.

2. **Vegetable Chips**:

   - Slice vegetables like sweet potatoes, beets, or zucchini thinly, toss with olive oil and seasoning, and bake until crispy. Homemade vegetable chips are a healthier alternative to store-bought varieties and are easy to make in large batches.

3. **Banana Oat Bars**:

   - Mash ripe bananas and mix with rolled oats, cinnamon, and your choice of add-ins such as nuts, seeds, or dried fruit. Press into a baking dish and bake until golden brown for a wholesome and budget-friendly snack option.

Budget-Friendly Snack Packs for On-the-Go Convenience

1. **DIY Trail Mix Packs**:

- Prepare individual snack packs containing a mix of nuts, seeds, dried fruit, and whole grain cereal. These pre-portioned packs are convenient for snacking on the go and can be customized to suit your taste preferences.

2. **Vegetable Sticks with Hummus**:

- Slice vegetables like carrots, celery, and bell peppers into sticks and portion into individual containers. Pair with single-serve packets of hummus for a nutritious and satisfying snack that's perfect for busy days.

3. **Hard-Boiled Eggs**:

- Hard-boiled eggs are a protein-rich snack that can be prepared in advance and enjoyed on the go. Pack them in individual containers with a sprinkle of salt and pepper for a quick and convenient snack option.

By incorporating these budget-friendly snack ideas into your meal planning routine, you can satisfy your cravings without overspending. Whether you're at home or on the go, these snacks are sure to keep you fueled and energized throughout the day without breaking the bank.

CHAPTER SEVEN

Desserts Without the Splurge

Indulging in dessert doesn't have to mean breaking the bank. With a little creativity and resourcefulness, you can satisfy your sweet tooth with delicious treats that won't put a strain on your budget. This guide presents lower-cost dessert recipes for satisfying sweet cravings, fruit-based desserts that are naturally sweet and inexpensive, and budget-friendly baking recipes with simple ingredients.

Lower-Cost Dessert Recipes for Satisfying Sweet Cravings

1. **Chocolate Peanut Butter Oat Bars**:

   - Ingredients:

     - Rolled oats

     - Peanut butter

     - Honey or maple syrup

     - Cocoa powder

     - Optional mix-ins: chocolate chips, chopped nuts, dried fruit

   - Instructions:

1.   In a mixing bowl, combine rolled oats, peanut butter, honey or maple syrup, and cocoa powder until well combined.

2.   Stir in optional mix-ins if desired.

3.   Press the mixture into a baking dish and refrigerate until set.

4.   Cut into bars and enjoy a satisfying and budget-friendly sweet treat.

2. **No-Bake Energy Bites**:

- Ingredients:
    - Rolled oats
    - Nut butter (e.g., peanut butter, almond butter)
    - Honey or maple syrup
    - Optional mix-ins: chocolate chips, shredded coconut, chia seeds
- Instructions:

1.   In a mixing bowl, combine rolled oats, nut butter, honey or maple syrup, and optional mix-ins until well combined.

2.   Roll the mixture into bite-sized balls and refrigerate until firm.

3.   Enjoy as a quick and convenient dessert or snack that's packed with energy-boosting ingredients.

Fruit-Based Desserts That Are Naturally Sweet and Inexpensive

1. **Baked Apples**:

- Ingredients:

  - Apples

  - Cinnamon

  - Honey or maple syrup (optional)

  - Granola or chopped nuts (optional)

- Instructions:

1. Preheat the oven to 375°F (190°C).

2. Core apples and place them in a baking dish.

3. Sprinkle cinnamon over the apples and drizzle with honey or maple syrup if desired.

4. Bake for 25-30 minutes or until apples are tender.

5. Serve hot with a sprinkle of granola or chopped nuts for added texture and flavor.

2. **Frozen Banana Bites**:

- Ingredients:

  - Bananas

  - Nut butter (e.g., peanut butter, almond butter)

- Dark chocolate

- Instructions:

1. Slice bananas into rounds and spread nut butter between two slices to make sandwiches.

2. Dip banana sandwiches into melted dark chocolate until fully coated.

3. Place chocolate-covered banana bites on a parchment-lined baking sheet and freeze until firm.

4. Enjoy straight from the freezer as a refreshing and naturally sweet dessert option.

Budget-Friendly Baking Recipes with Simple Ingredients

1. **Classic Banana Bread**:

   - Ingredients:

     - Ripe bananas

     - Flour

     - Sugar

     - Eggs

     - Baking soda

     - Optional mix-ins: chopped nuts, chocolate chips

- Instructions:

1. Preheat the oven to 350°F (175°C) and grease a loaf pan.

2. In a mixing bowl, mash ripe bananas and mix with sugar, eggs, and baking soda.

3. Gradually stir in flour until just combined, being careful not to overmix.

4. Fold in optional mix-ins if desired.

5. Pour batter into the prepared loaf pan and bake for 50-60 minutes or until a toothpick inserted into the center comes out clean.

6. Let cool before slicing and enjoying a classic and comforting dessert that's easy on the wallet.

2. **Simple Sugar Cookies**:

- Ingredients:
  - Flour
  - Sugar
  - Butter
  - Eggs
  - Baking powder
- Instructions:

1.   Preheat the oven to 350°F (175°C) and line a baking sheet with parchment paper.

2.   In a mixing bowl, cream together butter and sugar until light and fluffy.

3.   Beat in eggs one at a time, then stir in flour and baking powder until a dough forms.

4.   Roll dough into balls and place them on the prepared baking sheet.

5.   Flatten each ball with the bottom of a glass dipped in sugar.

6.   Bake for 8-10 minutes or until edges are lightly golden.

7.   Let cool before serving as a simple and budget-friendly sweet treat.

With these lower-cost dessert recipes, you can enjoy delicious sweets without overspending. Whether you prefer fruity treats, no-bake options, or classic baked goods, there's something for everyone to enjoy without breaking the bank.

CHAPTER EIGHT

Side Dishes That Won't Break the Bank

When planning meals, side dishes are often an essential component, providing balance, flavor, and nutritional value to the main course. However, side dishes don't have to be expensive to be delicious. This guide presents simple vegetable side dishes using affordable produce, budget-friendly whole grain and legume sides for balanced meals, and creative ways to add flavor to your side dishes without spending much.

Simple Vegetable Side Dishes Using Affordable Produce

1. **Roasted Vegetables**:

   - Ingredients:

     - Assorted vegetables (e.g., carrots, potatoes, broccoli, cauliflower)

     - Olive oil

     - Salt and pepper

     - Optional herbs and spices (e.g., garlic powder, thyme, rosemary)

   - Instructions:

1. Preheat the oven to 425°F (220°C).

2.   Chop vegetables into bite-sized pieces and toss with olive oil, salt, pepper, and optional herbs and spices.

3.   Spread vegetables in a single layer on a baking sheet.

4.   Roast in the preheated oven for 20-25 minutes or until vegetables are tender and caramelized.

5.   Serve hot as a flavorful and budget-friendly side dish.

2. **Sautéed Greens**:

- Ingredients:
    - Leafy greens (e.g., spinach, kale, Swiss chard)
    - Olive oil
    - Garlic, minced
    - Salt and pepper
- Instructions:

1.   Heat olive oil in a skillet over medium heat.

2.   Add minced garlic and sauté until fragrant.

3.   Add leafy greens to the skillet and cook until wilted.

4.   Season with salt and pepper to taste.

5.   Serve hot as a nutritious and affordable side dish.

Budget-Friendly Whole Grain and Legume Sides for Balanced Meals

1. **Quinoa Pilaf**:

   - Ingredients:

     - Quinoa

     - Vegetable broth or water

     - Assorted vegetables (e.g., bell peppers, onions, peas)

     - Olive oil

     - Salt and pepper

   - Instructions:

1. Rinse quinoa under cold water.

2. In a saucepan, heat olive oil over medium heat.

3. Add rinsed quinoa and toast for a few minutes until fragrant.

4. Stir in vegetable broth or water and bring to a boil.

5. Reduce heat, cover, and simmer for 15-20 minutes until quinoa is cooked and liquid is absorbed.

6. Fluff quinoa with a fork and stir in sautéed vegetables.

7.   Season with salt and pepper to taste and serve hot as a wholesome and budget-friendly side dish.

2. **Black Bean Salad**:

- Ingredients:
    - Canned black beans, drained and rinsed
    - Corn kernels (fresh, frozen, or canned)
    - Bell peppers, diced
    - Red onion, diced
    - Cilantro, chopped
    - Lime juice
    - Olive oil
    - Salt and pepper
- Instructions:

1.   In a large bowl, combine black beans, corn kernels, diced bell peppers, diced red onion, and chopped cilantro.

2.   Drizzle with lime juice and olive oil, and toss to combine.

3.   Season with salt and pepper to taste.

4.   Serve chilled or at room temperature as a flavorful and budget-friendly side dish.

Creative Ways to Add Flavor to Your Side Dishes Without Spending Much

1. **Herb Butter**:

   - Mix softened butter with chopped fresh herbs like parsley, thyme, or rosemary. Spread over cooked vegetables or grains for a burst of flavor.

2. **Citrus Zest**:

   - Grate the zest of lemons, limes, or oranges over cooked side dishes for a bright and zesty flavor boost.

3. **Spice Blends**:

   - Create your own spice blends using pantry staples like cumin, paprika, garlic powder, and onion powder. Sprinkle over roasted vegetables or grains for added depth of flavor.

By incorporating these simple and budget-friendly side dishes into your meals, you can enjoy delicious and balanced meals without overspending. With the right ingredients and a little creativity, you can elevate any meal without breaking the bank.

CHAPTER NINE

Eating Out and Socializing on a Budget

Maintaining a social life while adhering to a budget can seem challenging, especially when it comes to dining out and attending social events. However, with careful planning and smart choices, it's possible to enjoy socializing without overspending. This guide offers strategies for making healthy choices when dining out without breaking the bank, tips for navigating social events and special occasions on a budget, and advice on sticking to your budget while eating out with friends and family.

Strategies for Making Healthy Choices When Dining Out Without Overspending

1. **Research Menus in Advance**: Before heading to a restaurant, take a look at the menu online. Look for healthier options such as grilled or baked dishes, salads, and vegetable-based entrees. Planning ahead can help you make informed choices and avoid impulse decisions at the restaurant.

2. **Watch Portion Sizes**: Many restaurants serve oversized portions, which can lead to overeating and overspending. Consider splitting a meal with a friend or family member, or ask for a half portion if available. Alternatively, ask for a to-go box at the beginning of the meal and portion out half of your meal to take home for later.

3. **Choose Water or Unsweetened Beverages**: Beverages can significantly add to the cost of a meal, especially alcoholic drinks and sugary beverages. Opt for water or unsweetened beverages to save money and reduce calorie intake. If you're dining out with friends, suggest splitting a pitcher of water instead of ordering individual drinks.

Tips for Navigating Social Events and Special Occasions on a Budget

1. **Offer to Host Potluck Dinners**: Instead of dining out at a restaurant, suggest hosting a potluck dinner at home. Ask each guest to bring a dish to share, which not only reduces the cost for everyone but also adds variety to the meal. Hosting potluck dinners allows you to socialize with friends and family without overspending.

2. **Set a Spending Limit for Gifts**: Special occasions like birthdays and holidays often involve gift-giving, which can strain your budget. To avoid overspending, set a spending limit for gifts and consider creative and thoughtful alternatives such as homemade gifts or experiences rather than material items.

3. **Look for Free or Low-Cost Activities**: Socializing doesn't have to revolve around expensive meals or events. Look for free or low-cost activities such as picnics in the park, hiking, or attending community events and festivals. These activities

allow you to spend time with loved ones without breaking the bank.

How to Stick to Your Budget While Eating Out with Friends and Family

1. **Suggest Budget-Friendly Restaurants**: When making plans to eat out with friends or family, suggest restaurants that offer affordable options. Look for restaurants with lunch specials, happy hour deals, or discounts for large groups. Choosing budget-friendly restaurants helps ensure that everyone can enjoy the meal without overspending.

2. **Set Expectations in Advance**: Before dining out with friends or family, communicate your budgetary constraints and set expectations accordingly. Let them know that you're trying to stick to a budget and suggest alternatives such as sharing appetizers or desserts instead of ordering individual items. Open communication helps avoid awkwardness and ensures that everyone is on the same page.

3. **Practice Mindful Eating**: While dining out, practice mindful eating by paying attention to hunger cues and savoring each bite. Slow down and enjoy the conversation and company of friends and family rather than focusing solely on the food. By being mindful of your eating habits, you can avoid overordering and overspending.

By implementing these strategies and tips, you can enjoy dining out and socializing with friends and family without compromising your budget or health goals. With careful planning and smart choices, you can strike a balance between socializing and saving money.

CHAPTER TEN

Meal Planning and Prep for Low-Cost Eating

Eating on a budget doesn't have to mean sacrificing taste or nutrition. With effective meal planning and preparation strategies, you can enjoy delicious and affordable meals while saving both time and money. This guide offers practical tips for meal planning and grocery shopping on a budget, batch cooking and freezing meals to save money and time, and maximizing leftovers and reducing food waste to stretch your budget even further.

Practical Tips for Meal Planning and Grocery Shopping on a Budget

1. **Plan Your Meals Weekly**: Take some time each week to plan out your meals for the upcoming week. Consider your schedule, dietary preferences, and ingredients you already have on hand. Planning your meals in advance helps you avoid impulse purchases and reduces the likelihood of food waste.

2. **Make a Grocery List and Stick to It**: Before heading to the grocery store, make a list of the ingredients you'll need for your planned meals. Stick to your list while shopping to avoid unnecessary purchases. Consider using grocery apps or

websites to compare prices and find the best deals on essential items.

3. **Shop Seasonally and Locally**: Seasonal produce is often more affordable and fresher than out-of-season options. Visit local farmers' markets or look for sales and discounts at grocery stores to save money on fresh fruits and vegetables. Buying locally sourced ingredients can also support small businesses and reduce your environmental impact.

Batch Cooking and Freezing Meals to Save Money and Time

1. **Choose Versatile Ingredients**: When meal planning, choose versatile ingredients that can be used in multiple recipes. For example, a large batch of cooked grains like rice or quinoa can serve as the base for various meals throughout the week. Similarly, proteins like beans or chicken can be incorporated into different dishes.

2. **Cook in Bulk**: Dedicate a day or evening to batch cooking large quantities of food that can be portioned out and frozen for future meals. Cooked soups, stews, casseroles, and sauces are ideal candidates for batch cooking and freezing. Invest in freezer-safe containers or bags to store your meals efficiently.

3. **Label and Date**: When freezing meals, be sure to label each container or bag with the contents and date of preparation. This makes it easier to keep track of what you have on hand and ensures that older items are used before newer ones.

Maximizing Leftovers and Reducing Food Waste to Stretch Your Budget

1. **Repurpose Leftovers**: Get creative with leftovers by transforming them into new meals. For example, leftover roasted vegetables can be added to omelets or salads, while cooked grains can be turned into fried rice or grain bowls. Experiment with different flavor combinations to breathe new life into leftovers.

2. **Practice FIFO (First In, First Out)**: When organizing your refrigerator and pantry, follow the FIFO principle by placing older items at the front and newer items at the back. This helps ensure that older ingredients are used before they spoil, reducing food waste and saving money.

3. **Use Every Part of the Ingredient**: Don't discard edible parts of ingredients that are often overlooked, such as vegetable stems, herb stems, or meat bones. These can be used to make stocks, broths, and sauces, adding flavor to your meals while reducing waste.

By implementing these meal planning and preparation strategies, you can enjoy nutritious and budget-friendly meals while minimizing food waste and saving time in the kitchen. With a little planning and creativity, eating well on a budget is not only achievable but also enjoyable.

CHAPTER 11

31 DAYS MEAL PLAN

Day 1:

- Breakfast: Oatmeal with sliced bananas and a sprinkle of cinnamon.

- Lunch: Turkey and cheese sandwich on whole grain bread with lettuce and tomato.

- Dinner: Baked chicken thighs with roasted vegetables (carrots, bell peppers, and onions).

Day 2:

- Breakfast: Scrambled eggs with spinach and tomatoes, served with whole grain toast.

- Lunch: Tuna salad with mixed greens and whole wheat crackers.

- Dinner: Lentil soup with a side of steamed broccoli.

Day 3:

- Breakfast: Greek yogurt with sliced peaches and a sprinkle of granola.

- Lunch: Veggie stir-fry with tofu and brown rice.

- Dinner: Baked fish fillets with a squeeze of lemon, served with mashed sweet potatoes and green beans.

Day 4:

- Breakfast: Whole grain toast with almond butter and sliced apple.

- Lunch: Chickpea salad with cucumber, tomatoes, and a light vinaigrette dressing.

- Dinner: Turkey meatballs in marinara sauce, served over whole wheat spaghetti.

Day 5:

- Breakfast: Smoothie made with spinach, banana, almond milk, and a scoop of protein powder.

- Lunch: Egg salad sandwich with whole grain bread and lettuce.

- Dinner: Stir-fried shrimp with mixed vegetables and brown rice.

Day 6:

- Breakfast: Cottage cheese with diced pineapple and a sprinkle of cinnamon.

- Lunch: Quinoa and black bean salad with corn, bell peppers, and salsa.

- Dinner: Baked chicken drumsticks with roasted Brussels sprouts and quinoa.

Day 7:

- Breakfast: Whole grain waffles with sliced strawberries and a drizzle of honey.

- Lunch: Turkey and avocado wrap with lettuce and whole wheat tortilla.

- Dinner: Vegetable curry with chickpeas, served with brown rice.

Day 8:

- Breakfast: Oatmeal with sliced bananas and a sprinkle of cinnamon.

- Lunch: Lentil soup with diced carrots and celery.

- Dinner: Baked salmon with roasted asparagus and quinoa.

Day 9:

- Breakfast: Scrambled eggs with diced bell peppers and onions, served with whole grain toast.

- Lunch: Tuna salad with mixed greens and cherry tomatoes, dressed with balsamic vinaigrette.

- Dinner: Stir-fried tofu with broccoli and snap peas, served over brown rice.

Day 10:

- Breakfast: Greek yogurt with mixed berries and a sprinkle of granola.

- Lunch: Turkey and cheese sandwich on whole grain bread with lettuce and tomato.

- Dinner: Baked cod with lemon and herbs, served with roasted cauliflower and whole wheat couscous.

Day 11:

- Breakfast: Whole grain toast with mashed avocado and poached eggs.

- Lunch: Chickpea salad with cucumber, tomatoes, and a light vinaigrette dressing.

- Dinner: Turkey chili with kidney beans and diced vegetables, served with a side salad.

Day 12:

- Breakfast: Smoothie made with spinach, banana, almond milk, and a scoop of protein powder.

- Lunch: Veggie stir-fry with tofu and brown rice.

- Dinner: Baked chicken thighs with roasted vegetables (carrots, bell peppers, and onions).

Day 13:

- Breakfast: Cottage cheese with diced pineapple and a sprinkle of cinnamon.

- Lunch: Quinoa and black bean salad with corn, bell peppers, and salsa.

- Dinner: Baked fish fillets with a squeeze of lemon, served with mashed sweet potatoes and green beans.

Day 14:

- Breakfast: Whole grain waffles with sliced strawberries and a drizzle of honey.

- Lunch: Turkey and avocado wrap with lettuce and whole wheat tortilla.

- Dinner: Vegetable curry with chickpeas, served with brown rice.

Day 15:

- Breakfast: Oatmeal with sliced bananas and a sprinkle of cinnamon.

- Lunch: Turkey and cheese sandwich on whole grain bread with lettuce and tomato.

- Dinner: Lentil soup with a side of steamed broccoli.

Day 16:

- Breakfast: Scrambled eggs with spinach and tomatoes, served with whole grain toast.

- Lunch: Tuna salad with mixed greens and whole wheat crackers.

- Dinner: Baked chicken thighs with roasted vegetables (carrots, bell peppers, and onions).

Day 17:

- Breakfast: Greek yogurt with sliced peaches and a sprinkle of granola.

- Lunch: Veggie stir-fry with tofu and brown rice.

- Dinner: Baked fish fillets with a squeeze of lemon, served with mashed sweet potatoes and green beans.

Day 18:

- Breakfast: Whole grain toast with almond butter and sliced apple.

- Lunch: Chickpea salad with cucumber, tomatoes, and a light vinaigrette dressing.

- Dinner: Turkey meatballs in marinara sauce, served over whole wheat spaghetti.

Day 19:

- Breakfast: Smoothie made with spinach, banana, almond milk, and a scoop of protein powder.

- Lunch: Egg salad sandwich with whole grain bread and lettuce.

- Dinner: Stir-fried shrimp with mixed vegetables and brown rice.

Day 20:

- Breakfast: Cottage cheese with diced pineapple and a sprinkle of cinnamon.

- Lunch: Quinoa and black bean salad with corn, bell peppers, and salsa.

- Dinner: Baked chicken drumsticks with roasted Brussels sprouts and quinoa.

Day 21:

- Breakfast: Whole grain waffles with sliced strawberries and a drizzle of honey.

- Lunch: Turkey and avocado wrap with lettuce and whole wheat tortilla.

- Dinner: Vegetable curry with chickpeas, served with brown rice.

Day 22:

- Breakfast: Oatmeal with sliced bananas and a sprinkle of cinnamon.

- Lunch: Lentil soup with diced carrots and celery.

- Dinner: Baked salmon with roasted asparagus and quinoa.

Day 23:

- Breakfast: Scrambled eggs with diced bell peppers and onions, served with whole grain toast.

- Lunch: Tuna salad with mixed greens and cherry tomatoes, dressed with balsamic vinaigrette.

- Dinner: Stir-fried tofu with broccoli and snap peas, served over brown rice.

Day 24:

- Breakfast: Greek yogurt with mixed berries and a sprinkle of granola.

- Lunch: Turkey and cheese sandwich on whole grain bread with lettuce and tomato.

- Dinner: Baked cod with lemon and herbs, served with roasted cauliflower and whole wheat couscous.

Day 25:

- Breakfast: Whole grain toast with mashed avocado and poached eggs.

- Lunch: Chickpea salad with cucumber, tomatoes, and a light vinaigrette dressing.

- Dinner: Turkey chili with kidney beans and diced vegetables, served with a side salad.

Day 26:

- Breakfast: Smoothie made with spinach, banana, almond milk, and a scoop of protein powder.

- Lunch: Veggie stir-fry with tofu and brown rice.

- Dinner: Baked chicken thighs with roasted vegetables (carrots, bell peppers, and onions).

Day 27:

- Breakfast: Cottage cheese with diced pineapple and a sprinkle of cinnamon.

- Lunch: Quinoa and black bean salad with corn, bell peppers, and salsa.

- Dinner: Baked fish fillets with a squeeze of lemon, served with mashed sweet potatoes and green beans.

Day 28:

- Breakfast: Whole grain waffles with sliced strawberries and a drizzle of honey.

- Lunch: Turkey and avocado wrap with lettuce and whole wheat tortilla.

- Dinner: Vegetable curry with chickpeas, served with brown rice.

Day 29:

- Breakfast: Oatmeal with sliced bananas and a sprinkle of cinnamon.

- Lunch: Lentil soup with a side of steamed broccoli.

- Dinner: Baked chicken thighs with roasted vegetables (carrots, bell peppers, and onions).

Day 30:

- Breakfast: Scrambled eggs with spinach and tomatoes, served with whole grain toast.

- Lunch: Tuna salad with mixed greens and whole wheat crackers.

- Dinner: Baked salmon with roasted asparagus and quinoa.

Day 31:

- Breakfast: Greek yogurt with sliced peaches and a sprinkle of granola.

- Lunch: Veggie stir-fry with tofu and brown rice.

- Dinner: Turkey meatballs in marinara sauce, served over whole wheat spaghetti.

THE END